FIVE HOSPITALS
AND A
MEDICAL JOURNEY
THROUGH HELL

DON'T THINK THIS COULDN'T HAPPEN TO YOU

ROGER E. GUSSETT

ARCHWAY
PUBLISHING

Copyright © 2018 Roger E. Gussett.

All rights reserved. No part of this book may be used or reproduced by any means, graphic, electronic, or mechanical, including photocopying, recording, taping or by any information storage retrieval system without the written permission of the author except in the case of brief quotations embodied in critical articles and reviews.

Archway Publishing books may be ordered through booksellers or by contacting:

Archway Publishing
1663 Liberty Drive
Bloomington, IN 47403
www.archwaypublishing.com
1 (888) 242-5904

Because of the dynamic nature of the Internet, any web addresses or links contained in this book may have changed since publication and may no longer be valid. The views expressed in this work are solely those of the author and do not necessarily reflect the views of the publisher, and the publisher hereby disclaims any responsibility for them.

Any people depicted in stock imagery provided by Getty Images are models, and such images are being used for illustrative purposes only. Certain stock imagery © Getty Images.

ISBN: 979-8-6709-3130-4 (sc)
ISBN: 978-1-4808-6279-1 (e)

Library of Congress Control Number: 2018905298

Print information available on the last page.

Archway Publishing rev. date: 06/11/2018

Contents

Chapter 1	Her youth couldn't have been worse. Then she became an ovarian cancer survivor at the age twenty	1
Chapter 2	Terry the entrepreneur	3
Chapter 3	The effects of radiation damage to her health was gradual over many years involving multiple organ functions, especially her immune, gastrointestinal, and renal systems	7
Chapter 4	Fat malabsorption resulted in multiple vitamin deficiencies including vitamin A. If left undiagnosed, this condition could lead to permanent blindness	10
Chapter 5	Peritoneal dialysis in 2004 and a kidney transplant in 2006	12
Chapter 6	The intestinal obstruction and resection completed in 2013 at Rochester including complications with "third spacing"	14
Chapter 7	Further complications after leaving Rochester with multiple hospital admissions in Naples. Terry's vacation that never happened	21
Chapter 8	The return to Toledo to find out what went wrong and an intestinal re-obstruction surgery completed in Cleveland. The only successful "third spacing" event and out of the hospital in 1 week	25
Chapter 9	Changes in Obama care result in Terry's removal from total parenteral nutrition	30

Chapter 10 The third surgery in three years a successful spinal abscess surgery in Cleveland, but a disastrous aftercare including another "third spacing" incident and the imposition of a rectal hose eventually leading to her removal of life support. 37

Chapter 11 My sense of disbelief and my attempt to assemble information needed to understand what went wrong by retrieving Terry's medical reports... 46

Chapter 12 My complaints issued to Medicare, The Commission, and the State Medical Board who stonewalled me hoping I would just go away .55

PREFACE

There are some people in this world that go through life with merely a blemish. Others such as Terry, my companion for over thirty years, endured hardships from the very early years of her life and continued to experience those hardships throughout her lifetime. This is a true story of one of those unfortunate, truly remarkable individuals, that despite all life's misfortunes, became a successful entrepreneur. Her father, who initially was a successful businessman, due to a business failure committed suicide while Terry was the tender age of nine-years old. Her mother then became an alcoholic, and her grandmother assumed the responsibility to raise her. At the age of twenty, Terry became a victim of ovarian cancer and was not expected to live. Despite her dire prognosis, she survived radiation treatments but was left with life long side effects that plagued her throughout her lifetime. Even still, her entrepreneurialism allowed her to proceed through life to experience the joy of achievements of many occupations. Her biggest achievements were as an interior decorator, which led her to become a builder of homes, and ultimately to become a developer. The main scope of this book centers around her medical long-term effects from radiation treatments that, over many years, resulted in a gradual deterioration in her health. In medicine, it exposes the successes, but it also reveals some of the inexcusable events that led to her death. The book exposes doctor's and hospital's differences in opinions of how to address the same medical calamities leading to very different results. In addition, at issue is the indifference by a State Medical Board and various agencies to the dilemma. We together traveled thousands of medical miles hoping for a resolution that never came. My profession was a veterinarian small animal practitioner, owner of my own small animal business for nearly forty years. Prior to that, I had been a member of the United States Army Veterinary Corp serving in multiple capacities, as food inspection, large and small animal disease and treatment, and prevention. Through my medical experience and training, I was able to assist Terry in her many struggles. This story has been presented factually to the best of my ability as to remembering events and timelines, as we together traveled through "Five Hospitals and A Medical Journey Through Hell".

Acknowledgment

I would like to express my thanks and appreciation to all of Terry's friends that maintained contact with Terry or accompanied us through our medical journey spanning thousands of miles. In particular, thanks to Susan who visited Terry soon after Terry's initial obstruction surgery in the fall of 2013. Then, two months later, Susan made airline arrangement for herself to return to Rochester and assist Terry's return to Toledo. Finally, I wish to thank Kathy, Terry's sister-in-law, and Sue for accompanying me to Terry's final visit, prior to my decision to remove Terry from life support.

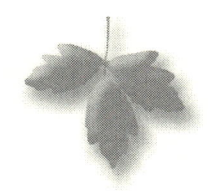

CHAPTER I

This story is about a beautiful woman both inside and out who despite a life of many adverse events was able to achieve what most people would have only dreamed of. At the tender age of nine, Terry's father a successful business man, committed suicide as a result of a business failure. Ultimately her mother became an alcoholic, and her grandmother became responsible for raising her. She was a free-spirited young girl, a tom-boy at heart, who at a young age was more likely to be involved in sports with the guys. She was often involved in local sandlot baseball games, never really interested in the kinds of things most girls were, such as playing with dolls. Surrounded by three other brothers, it was hard for her to be involved in anything other than sports. As a teenager, she had worked several stints at fast food restaurants to earn money with the hopes of one day going to college.

Then at the age of nineteen, Terry married and soon moved to Louisiana to join her husband in the military. While there she had the unfortunate fate of becoming an ovarian cancer victim. The prognosis was extremely poor, and she was not expected to survive, as the cancer had spread to her abdominal cavity. She was transferred for treatment to the Anderson Cancer Institute in Houston, Texas. The treatment in 1970 was radiation, as current treatments were not yet available. The ill effects of radiation's long-term use had not been established, and valuable organs were not well protected. The doctors knew little about how to cure ovarian cancer, especially when it had metastasized throughout the abdominal cavity. As it turned out, the course of treatment allowed her to survive. Soon after radiation treatments, Terry began to experience side effects such as chronic diarrhea and severe painful, abdominal spasms. The chronic diarrhea continued the rest of her life, as radiation damaged her large bowel's essential function to reabsorb water.

Years later, Terry began experiencing vomiting attacks, initially occurring several times a year, but gradually over time, these attacks became much worse. She learned through experience to consume a liquid diet, allowing her bowel to rest and recover. She also ate small meals and avoided foods that may have caused her problems in the past. Painful abdominal spasms from severe straining episodes accompanied the diarrhea, when it became most severe. Despite the chronic diarrhea and other side effects, Terry gradually gained her weight back six months following radiation treatments. Her strength, vitality, and overall health returned to normal.

After her husband completed military service, Terry and her husband returned to Toledo. The readjustment to civilian life had not been easy for Terry and her husband, and there had been constant turmoil. In addition, Terry's near life-ending medical issues had weighed heavily on her. Their relationship soon ended in divorce. Terry's past relationships with her grandmother had been a monumental influence in Terry's life, establishing Terry's positive attitude and independence. These very important traits were paramount in her overcoming her earlier hardships. Terry soon began to plan her life. She decided to obtain certification for a medical radiology technician degree, so as to become employed at a local hospital. She enjoyed the work, but after several years of working in the field, it became routine and boring. In addition, the occupation required some night work which she didn't care for.

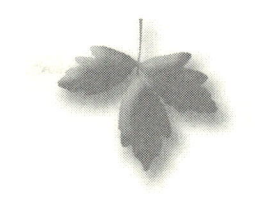

CHAPTER II

Then in 1978, Terry met and married Rudy. While married to Rudy, Terry decided to branch out in a variety of employment fields, which included painting, wallpapering, and buying and selling plants. These jobs all required long hours, especially since she lacked the necessary knowledge and experience to successfully fulfill these tasks. Terry spent hours reading, so as to digest all important information, so she could be the best at what ever endeavor she pursued. These jobs were entrepreneurial, since she was not one to work for other people. Terry was independent and enjoyed the freedom of establishing when and how she would work those long hours. She began to develop other outside interests, such as cooking and antiques. Cooking became a special interest at holidays and she spent hours developing new dishes for family members.

Rudy introduced Terry to the sport of tennis. He had played tennis for several years as a member of Shadow Valley Tennis Club and the Toledo Tennis Club. Rudy began spending a lot of time improving Terry's tennis game. She quickly became an avid tennis player and achieved a 4.0 skill rating. Later, she entered and won several tennis tournaments.

Then in 1985, Terry and Rudy divorced. At the time, both Terry and Rudy were members of the Toledo Tennis Club. I met Rudy shortly after their divorce. Rudy and I had been introduced through a mutual tennis friend at the Toledo Tennis Club. We soon began playing tennis several times a week and joined a league sponsored by that club. Both of us had played other sports, deciding this was a sport for a lifetime that could fit into our busy work schedules. Despite the divorce, Terry had retained her membership at the Toledo Tennis Club.

Soon after the divorce, Rudy invited me to a party that would forever change my life. Rudy informed me that the party was a divorce party arranged by his ex-wife, Terry. Despite the divorce, they had maintained an amicable relationship. Since they had recently divorced, I knew Rudy still had feelings for her. I had, myself, recently divorced, a victim of a very demanding occupation-veterinary medicine. I found Terry to be very attractive and enthusiastic. I was attracted to her immediately, but I was not yet ready for another relationship.

Then months later, while at my veterinary clinic, I was informed a client had brought in an injured squirrel. It so happened that the client was Terry, whom I had met at Rudy's divorce party. I recognized her immediately. The squirrel was in sad shape, as it had two broken legs. I informed Terry it would be most humane to put it to sleep. I had not expected her to consider treatment. Instead, she asked whether or not I could fix the squirrel's legs. I told her it would be difficult and time consuming, but that I would try. I also informed her it would be $300. I was shocked when she asked me to do my best. The surgery consisted of employing two, tiny stainless-steel intramedullary pins in the femurs of the affected squirrel. Completed surgical time was three hours. The surgery was successful, and complete healing occurred eight weeks later. Upon returning for the squirrel's eight-week recheck, Terry informed me she was going to release the squirrel back into its natural habitat. She also informed me that she lived just down the street from my veterinary clinic.

One month later, while playing tennis with her ex-husband

Rudy at the Toledo Tennis Club, I happened to observe Terry playing tennis with some of her friends. She appeared to be a good player, so I asked whether she would be my mixed doubles partner in our club tournament. We entered the tournament, and soon became inseparable. Soon after, we moved in together.

At the time, Terry was working for a builder and was assisting in construction and interior decorating. She was very talented at furniture selection matching different color combinations with flooring, such as tile and carpet. She eventually decided to open her own interior decorating business. It was not long before clients were at her place of business asking for her input on interior design and furniture selection. Her expertise was so in demand that she was asked to assist with the Parade of Homes, a local home display event that featured some of the best builders in the area

Five years later, Terry decided she wanted to close her interior decorating business. The long hours and stress of the interior decorating business, plus her chronic health problems, forced her to consider other occupations. She had no retirement nor disability insurance, and chronic health problems continued to plague her. She became unsure of how long she could remain in business for herself and began to consider other occupations.

Government employment was considered. There she could receive sick leave, as well as the additional benefits of health insurance and retirement. She knew a lot of people who worked for the county, so she sent in her résumé for employment. Her employment was accepted, so she made arrangements to close the interior decorating business. Terry's new job was at the county treasurer's office. This job was a perfect fit for her at the time, since it allowed routine and regular hours of nine to five Monday through Friday, with free time on Saturdays and Sundays. Terry had plenty of time to enjoy tennis and other interests she previously could not participate in, due to the demands associated with working for herself. Through the county, Terry was able to develop new contacts that could help in future endeavors. Her work at the county also provided some insight into financial transactions and tax knowledge. She loved her work at the county treasurer's office, but eventually she left due to failing health and was placed on disability.

After several years of disability, Terry decided she needed something more to fulfill her life. She began working part time out of her home on different projects. From past experience working with local builders, as an interior decorator, Terry had met Dick Moses, a prominent developer in the Toledo area. She had always wanted to build a house, so Dick assisted her in the construction of a new home. From there nothing was too difficult for Terry. Soon after, and with no assistance, Terry constructed her own first house. After building several homes for individuals, she formed her own construction company, Avalon Homes. Despite her reoccurring medical difficulties, she worked at her own pace and initiated a residential development in which she bought and sold lots. She also assisted several lot purchasers in the construction of their new homes. Though unable to physically become involved, Terry was the brains behind the design and construction of her own residential development.

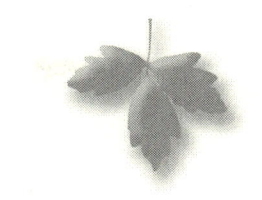

CHAPTER III

Her medical problems continued to daunt her, however. It became apparent that the side effects of years of radiation, coupled with her advancing age, were taking its toll. Terry's diarrhea, although present since the age of twenty-one, began to wear her down. It was not uncommon for her to go to the bathroom as many as twenty times a day. Present in her stool were tiny droplets of oil, evidence of fat malabsorption, which when she became older, emerged as symptoms of fat-soluble vitamin deficiencies. Some of the protein and vitamin deficiencies that in earlier years were not apparent suddenly surfaced. Over time, the radiation gradually reduced her intestinal tracts ability to assimilate nutrients exposing nutrient deficiencies. She began to lose muscle mass appearing malnourished, and with it, lost her general well-being. These deficiencies had never been addressed by physicians earlier in her medical life, prior to the actual onset of symptoms of disease.

Dehydration had always been an issue for Terry. She always had electrolyte containers and slept with a large two-quart ball jar, so as to rehydrate herself at night when getting up to go to the bathroom. While in transit, it was not uncommon for Terry not to make it to a bathroom, due to the explosive intestinal spasms that would sometimes occur. She would laugh about it because she knew I was embarrassed and thought someone might see her, as she stooped suddenly along a roadside. It was not uncommon for her to soil her underwear, as she couldn't quite make it to a restroom.

Periodically, she would have extreme vomiting attacks-"dry heaves", that would last hours and sometimes days at a time. Fortunately, these vomiting attacks earlier in her youth only occurred several times a year, but as she became older, they occurred more often. Terry would often not eat for several days, only consuming liquids, until the obstruction or inflammation would by itself resolve. If that didn't work, she would spend several days in a hospital on intravenous fluids. Because she had learned to eat smaller meals more often, and avoided foods that had previously created problems, Terry had been able to prevent hospitalizations that could otherwise have compounded her misery. Her abilities to understand her vomiting issues and dehydration, were especially noteworthy. My medical background helped give her some insight into her problems. For years, doctors were not fully aware of what Terry faced on a day to day basis, nor were they seemingly aware of future problems.

When I first met Terry, she was thirty-eight years old. She confided in me doctors stated her vomiting attacks were due to radiation enteritis acquired through radiation treatments for ovarian cancer, when she was twenty years-old. From her symptoms and past medical history, I suggested that there might be more involved than what doctors had been telling her. The irregularity of her vomiting attacks, unrelated to ingestion of food, might suggest additional causes for her intermittent vomiting. I stated she might have adrenal insufficiency, as radiation exposure to her abdomen could affect all body organs in that region. I reminded her that the adrenal gland could be affected, and adrenal insufficiency could be easily corrected by a simple once a day treatment of the drug, Florinef. This drug could be a replacement hormone for a steroid depleted by past radiation treatments.

Adrenal insufficiency had become a more commonly diagnosed disease in veterinary medicine due to improved testing and awareness, especially in dogs. The disease was associated with intermittent vomiting and occasionally diarrhea of waxing and waning nature. The disease was often difficult to diagnosis because other diseases might often appear similar. Also, diseases that involved vomiting were often treated in hospitals with saline, resulting in a temporary reprieve from the symptoms. I convinced her to see an endocrinologist in Cleveland for consultation. Terry obtained records from her hospital in Toledo located near her home and made an appointment with Cleveland Hospital #4 specifically to inquire about adrenal insufficiency. Terry was aware of her earlier diagnosis, radiation enteritis, but we wanted to know if she could be dealing with two problems instead of just one. Upon completion and review of her radiographs, the doctor in Cleveland was sure of his decision. Terry had radiation enteritis and he didn't feel it was necessary for further testing. So, no adrenal testing was completed.

Years later in 2004, Terry lost kidney function and was placed on dialysis. Then in 2006, she had a kidney transplant performed. Her kidney transplant was performed at Toledo Hospital #1 but doctors never questioned her adrenal gland function, even though its close proximity to the kidney. Then several years later, nausea and vomiting issues continued to surface gradually becoming more frequent. So, at my insistence, Terry again requested Toledo Hospital #1 do the adrenal test. Her test revealed the lowest normal limits. Despite a patient that physically appeared to have adrenal insufficiency, and a patient who had prior radiation exposure to the abdomen with symptoms of intermittent nausea and vomiting, doctors did not consider the possibility of a false negative test. Thus, lack of treatment could have spared her years of discomfort for intermittent nausea and vomiting. It wasn't until the spring of 2015, after recovering from an intestinal re-obstruction at the Cleveland Hospital #4, adrenal insufficiency was finally addressed.

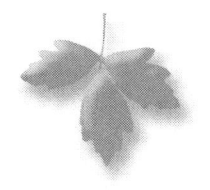

CHAPTER IV

Over time, an additional problem became apparent. Her chronic diarrhea with fat malabsorption led to fat-soluble vitamin deficiencies. Terry and I came home one night after going out to eat, and I noticed she was fumbling around the door knob trying to gain entry. It wasn't yet night time, so I asked if she was having problems with her eyesight. She said only at night, that her day vision was normal. I informed her that inability to absorb fat could lead to fat-soluble vitamin deficiencies including vitamin A. I had remembered as a teenager in high school, and later while in veterinary school, that vitamin A deficiency was a cause for night blindness. I suggested she see an ophthalmologist. She proceeded to contact several local ophthalmologists. Both considered vitamin A deficiency IMPOSSIBLE, since they had never diagnosed it, assuring her that it was a disease of impoverished countries. Despite the fact that Terry had presented the doctors with her symptoms, including chronic diarrhea with oil droplets, both ophthalmologists declined to do a simple blood test that would have easily diagnosed her problem.

Fast forward six months later, Terry and I were in Florida for a short vacation. Her vision was becoming increasingly worse. We happened to run into a tennis friend at the Tennis Club of Fort Lauderdale that was going to Miami for an eye exam. He had been diagnosed at the Bascom Palmer Eye Institute in Miami, Florida, for a rare form of glaucoma undiagnosed by doctors in his New Jersey area. Terry's eye sight had progressively worsened following her earlier eye exams in Toledo, and our friend had raved about Bascom Palmer stating it was world renowned. I suggested Terry make an appointment, and we would accompany our friend to Bascom Palmer Eye Institute. Armed with Terry's personal history including her symptoms of night blindness, within 30 minutes of the appointment, a young resident came back with blood test results for vitamin A stating Terry was indeed severely deficient in vitamin A. The doctor stated that had Terry continued undiagnosed, she would have become irreversibly blind. The doctor then prescribed a form of vitamin A injectable in a sustained release that was given monthly. It took two weeks for her vision to gradually return to normal. Shortly after returning from Bascom Palmer Eye Institute, Terry made a follow up appointment with Toledo Hospital #1. The doctors there found additional fat-soluble vitamin deficiencies. They made adjustments to her treatment by the addition of MCT oil to assist absorption of fats, as well as the vitamins. She continued to use the injectable vitamin A treatment for several more years until the company removed it from the market stating lack of sufficient demand. When Terry could no longer get the injectable vitamin A, she was forced to double the minimum daily requirement of oral vitamin A and consume it with MCT oil for absorption. This was to be continued for the rest of her life.

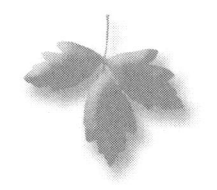

CHAPTER V

Then in 2004, Terry began to experience further problems, as her kidneys began to fail. She was placed on peritoneal dialysis. She hated this treatment, as it confined her forcing her to go to a clinic several times a week several hours a day. While on dialysis, she was placed on a donor list to receive a new kidney. She waited nearly two years before receiving a kidney. She had bypassed two earlier kidneys-one a prisoner that could have other problems as HIV or hepatitis, and the other kidney due to advanced age of the donor. On the very day Terry's new kidney became available, she had been hospitalized for a blood clot, while on peritoneal dialysis. She was very fortunate to receive a kidney taken from a teenager killed in an auto accident. The Toledo Hospital #1 did a miraculous job of titrating the balance between correcting the clot and still completing the renal transplant in 2006. I commend the doctors exceptional work.

After receiving her new kidney, Terry gradually over several months returned to a state of reasonably good health, with renewed strength and vitality. Much of her severe malnutrition from the kidney disease had been corrected with her weight returning to near normal. The doctors prescribed an immunosuppressant drug, tacrolimus, to prevent rejection of her new kidney. She began biking and playing tennis again. She still continued having diarrhea and occasional vomiting episodes, but nothing more than prior to the transplant. Bouts of anemia associated with poor assimilation of protein and iron also continued to plague her from time to time, as it had in her past. Her intestinal tracts ability to absorb nutrients had not yet been impaired. Her weight rarely fluctuated much through that time period maintaining a weight on average about 105 pounds. Terry did quite well from 2006, her kidney transplant, until 2013, the year of her intestinal obstruction.

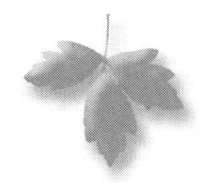

CHAPTER VI

Then, in May of 2013, a more serious problem surfaced. We had been vacationing in Florida when Terry began experiencing intermittent vomiting attacks that became more frequent and unremitting than prior attacks. She tried unsuccessfully to eat and hold down solid food. What was more alarming was liquids were being regurgitated as well. She had hoped her problems would resolve, as they had so many times before, by consuming only liquids while allowing her bowel to rest and recover. This time was different. Her inability to retain water resulted in increasing dehydration. We left Florida in early May 2013 to return to Toledo Hospital #1, where her kidney transplant surgery had been performed. She was administered intravenous fluids and appeared to be recovering. Terry and I discussed her condition as worsening and the need for possible intestinal surgery in the near future. We decided to contact a surgeon at Rochester Hospital #2 at the end of June 2013 for consultation, just in case surgery became necessary. We reasoned that the Rochester Hospital #2 would have more expertise in dealing with the unusual, such as radiation disease and its ancillary problems. During the early summer months, Terry's gastrointestinal issues continue to be up and down.

Then in August, Terry was readmitted to Toledo Hospital #1, where tests revealed she had an intestinal obstruction that necessitated surgical intervention. The doctors at Toledo Hospital #1 initiated intravenous fluid therapy as well as TPN, total parenteral nutrition. The TPN intravenous fluid had many ingredients for life preserving nutrition, such as vitamins, minerals, fats, amino acids, and carbohydrates. This therapy could allow a person like Terry to stay alive for a long period of time, despite being incapable of ingesting food. There were multiple side effects, such as liver disease, bone disease, infections, and others that she needed to remain vigilant while on this therapy. Monitoring was imperative. It took us several weeks to complete the necessary information to gain admittance to Rochester Hospital #2. All necessary steps were finalized and Rochester Hospital #2 and Toledo Hospital #1 made arrangements to transfer Terry to Rochester. Terry was transferred there by ambulance for the six-hour drive. Myself, and my companion "Snooter", my little 35# boston terrier, beagle-cross, followed Terry's ambulance by automobile.

Thus, began thousands of miles to and from multiple hospitals over the next three years, eventually ending in Terry's untimely removal from life support. Upon arrival at Rochester Hospital #2, I took residence at a motel directly across the street from where her post-operative care was to be administered. Terry was in a state of malnutrition, as she had been incapable of eating and drinking over the prior three weeks. Rochester Hospital #2 maintained Terry on TPN, and hospital personnel prepared her for what was to be a five-hour surgical procedure. The surgery included removal of the obstructed small bowel, as well as her colon. Much of her additional bowel removal was to prevent future obstructions, as radiation gradually over years had resulted in shrinkage and thickening, incapable of proper bowel function. Following surgery, the surgeon informed us that Terry had retained 135 centimeters of bowel. He defined this as having short bowel disease. He was unsure if that would be sufficient bowel to permit oral absorption of nutrients to maintain health and body mass. This meant the possibility she might have to be maintained on TPN for the rest of her life.

Following surgery, she spent approximately one week at an intensive care unit for follow up care. Post-surgically, she had been administered both Lasix, a diuretic to prevent fluid accumulation, and albumin, an essential blood protein that maintains fluid within the blood vessels. She was prescribed certain foods to eat and a dietary protein-vitamin supplement, Nutren, she was to take daily. When Terry left the intensive care unit, she was doing quite well. She was eating well and had begun an exercise routine, walking up and down the hallways several times a day improving rapidly. She was in pain, of course, but otherwise in good spirits. I remember some of her slurred speech and her inability to recall events. She also talked about events that were unassociated with the current time and place. I suggested to the doctors that these misgivings were probably associated with the narcotics used for pain. The nurses at Rochester Hospital #2 were excellent, and Terry was able to maintain the same nurse several days in succession, unlike some of the other hospitals she had visited.

Soon after leaving the intensive care unit, I noticed that Terry's arms, legs, and torso were beginning to accumulate excessive fluid. Both her appetite and exercise tolerance had declined dramatically. I knew that accumulation of fluid to this degree was very unhealthy. Much of her fluid was wasted, as it had accumulated outside her circulatory system into the pleural and peritoneal cavities, a condition termed "third spacing". Excessive fluid outside the circulatory system can suppress valuable organ function and compress blood vessels. The main purposes of intravenous fluids are electrolyte maintenance, blood pressure and hydration. I could see a direct correlation between her decreasing appetite and exercise tolerance to the amount of fluid she had begun to accumulate.

I discussed this subject with the surgeon. I suggested he needed to decrease the volume of intravenous fluid or eliminate it, and initiate the use of a diuretic, such as Lasix. I also suggested continuing the use of Lasix on an as needed basis to control the fluid. This would allow her to regain her appetite and enable her to exercise again. Immediately following surgery, she had been doing quite well. I stated the "third spacing" event could result in fluid entering her abdominal cavity, resulting in suture failure and his obstruction surgery to re-obstruct. The surgeon concurred he also was concerned about that. I exclaimed doctors not addressing this very important issue were defeating the very elements necessary for her recovery-appetite and exercise. The one thing Terry needed the most was to be able to ingest high biological protein food sources for a short time, so as to accumulate the blood protein albumin so as to reverse loss of fluid from her circulatory system. A patient whose weight had been bogged down with fluids some 30% to 40% more than normal would NOT feel much like eating or exercising. My advice fell on deaf ears. Doctors refused to use Lasix to control her over hydration on the premise that it could compromise her kidney transplant. My retort was that by not controlling the fluid, they were compromising her LIFE!

As swelling of her arms, legs, and torso became more apparent, Terry began to experience shortness of breath. She became so short of breath it was difficult for her to get up and down from the commode. She began to hyperventilate. Soon after, the doctors made the decision to send her to the intensive care unit, where they proceeded to use large needles to drain fluid from the pleural and peritoneal cavities. Terry explained these procedures as excruciatingly painful. Surprisingly, in the intensive care unit, after completing their needle draws, the doctors administered diuretics such as Lasix to remove additional fluid. This made absolutely no sense, as on the one hand they were telling Terry and I diuretics could compromise her one kidney, and while on the other hand, they were now administering those very drugs.

This was Terry's first experience with "third spacing", whereby intravenous fluid administered leaves the circulatory system to collect in body cavities such as the pleural and peritoneal cavities but could collect anywhere. This author is aware of different causes for "third spacing", but for this article focus will be on surgery, hypoproteinemia and the subsequent development of "third spacing". Fluid collection in body cavities are for all practical purposes wasted fluid and can be harmful. Patients malnourished with inadequate protein stores subjected to surgery are especially vulnerable to "third spacing". All of a sudden there is a surge in demand for the protein albumin for healing at surgical sites, which then lowers blood albumin. Albumin is necessary to retain fluid within the circulatory system and serves as an important factor in fluid homeostasis. Important sources of albumin are high biological proteins such as meat, eggs, milk, and milk by products such as cheese. In order for oral consumption to occur there must be a willing and ABLE patient. When the patient is laden with so much fluid, as to be noticeably apparent in their arms, legs, and torso as Terry, food and exercise becomes nearly intolerable.

Upon leaving the intensive care unit, doctors repeated what had gotten her in trouble originally. They continued administering intravenous fluid daily, whereupon over days fluid gradually accumulated in much the same pattern as before. Her arms, legs and torso became severely swollen. Her appetite and exercise tolerance were gone. Her breathing became labored again, as fluid filled her pleural and peritoneal cavities, and of course the doctors carted her away to the intensive care unit for a second time to repeat what they had done before. I had been living in a motel for over a month unsure if she could ever recover. I couldn't see a light at the end of the tunnel. I was constantly arguing with the doctors, as they kept repeating the same treatment over and over again. It was a roller coaster ride, first we were up then we were down. It was an exercise in futility.

While in her hospital rooms, Terry had talked to patients that stated some patients had been hospitalized at the Rochester Hospital #2 for years. As difficult as it was, I informed Terry I was going back to Toledo. The stress had become too much for me. When I left, I was unsure if I would ever see her alive again. When I returned to Toledo, I called her every day hoping my leaving would spur the doctors into altering their method of treatment. She was sent to an intensive care unit two or three more times after I left. Then, after returning from the intensive care unit for the last time, Terry made the statement, "why do these doctors insist on continually filling me up with so much fluid whereby I feel like an over inflated basketball". She couldn't understand their lack of flexibility. She exclaimed doctors should have to endure what she experienced to gain a better understanding how it affects their patients. Terry sounded strong, but I could tell she was very depressed at what was happening to her over and over again.

I suggested Terry try a different tactic. SHE needed to be the one to inform doctors SHE was requesting diuretics necessary to control the excess fluid accumulation, despite any risk to her one kidney. I further suggested SHE ask doctors to reduce the amount of fluid being maintained or eliminating it altogether. Finally, I asked Terry to try to remember how well she had felt following surgery, before doctors had allowed fluid to accumulate in her arms, legs and torso. I had remembered Terry's good appetite, and the many times she and I had walked up and down the hallways at Rochester Hospital #2. The doctors wouldn't listen to US before. Now, after nearly two months would they listen to HER now!

After our discussion, Terry summoned the doctors in charge of her case. They had a discussion amongst themselves. The nephrologist in charge of her case was relieved of her duty. A new nephrologist was placed in charge of her treatment. It had been almost two months of hospitalization, and Terry was hoping it would end. The doctor in charge made changes to control the amount of fluid delivered and included the use of diuretics. I received word she began feeling better almost immediately. From her voice I could hear strength. Soon after, I left for Florida to establish residency. I stayed in touch, as Terry expected to return to Toledo shortly. Several weeks later, I finally got the word Terry was given a date of release from the hospital. Much of the excess fluid had dissipated, and she felt like eating and exercising again. I was elated at the news. Terry's good friend, Susan, said she would assist Terry with the airline tickets, including picking her up at the Rochester Hospital #2 and taking her back to Toledo.

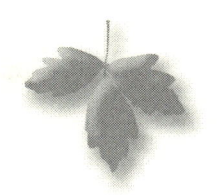

CHAPTER VII

It was late fall of 2013 when Terry finally arrived in Toledo. I could tell that something wasn't right in her voice. Soon after arrival, she notified me she had been admitted to Toledo Hospital #1 with an infection. The doctors treated her with antibiotics and fluids, and after several days, she was released. Upon leaving the hospital, a doctor suggested Terry begin a series of hyperbaric treatments that he thought might help bowel nutrient absorption by increasing oxygen to the lining of the intestinal tract. He theorized it might help her immune system as well. The term I believe he quoted Terry was neo-vascularization, as to the formation of new blood vessels to the intestinal lining. Terry underwent two to three months of hyperbaric treatments with questionable results. The side effects of hyperbaric treatments resulted in cataract formation six months after completion. Much later in 2015, her vision became so impaired Terry elected cataract removal.

In early December 2013, after recovering from the infections at Toledo Hospital #1, and completing the hyperbaric treatments, Terry began complaining about back pain doctors diagnosed as a kidney infection. The antibiotics dispensed didn't remove her pain. The doctors then x-rayed her back and spine and discovered a fractured rib. She was dispensed medication that seemed to improve her recovery for several months. She continued to complain about intermittent bone pain in early 2014. Finally, her bone pain became increasingly unbearable, so the doctors performed additional x-rays of her back and spine. They reported that new x-rays revealed that Terry had multiple foci involving the ribs, that to doctors indicated malignancy. The doctors then made an appointment for a surgical biopsy. Terry was a basket case, since she felt she had acquired cancer for the second time, albeit a different cell-type. Terry confided in me. I told her something just didn't seem right. Three months earlier the radiologist had diagnosed a fracture and now her condition was cancer!

Terry's sister by a prior marriage, Nancy, and I decided to do our own research. We were both aware of Terry's use of TPN. Nancy beat me to the punch by identifying metabolic bone disease, as a problem for TPN patients. I then researched multiple articles concerning metabolic bone disease associated with chronic TPN usage. I called Nancy with the good news, that I felt she was in fact correct. I was in Florida at the time, and suggested Terry call her radiologist. I told Terry it may not have been the same radiologist who viewed her original x-rays. I advised she explain to this recent radiologist that their radiology department had completed x-rays several months earlier suggesting a fractured rib. I also told her to inform the radiologist Terry had a friend who suggested a review of the original x-rays for comparison. Finally, I suggested she inform the radiologist of her prolonged TPN usage. Then, Terry was to suggest that she might have developed metabolic bone disease from chronic TPN usage, that ultimately may have led to her original fracture. Less than twenty-four hours later, the radiologist informed Terry he had canceled her biopsy. He explained to her that metabolic bone disease was indeed present and had resulted in multiple fractured ribs. Terry stated that five to seven ribs were involved. She was dispensed several nutritional drugs, as well as Calcitriol, and ordered to reduce TPN usage from five days a week, to three or four days a week. For the next several months,

Terry was maintained on multiple pain medications to alleviate the discomfort from her painful rib fractures.

Late in the spring of 2014 Terry decided to accompany a friend, Dick Moses, by airline to Naples, Florida, to visit me. I told her not to come if she hadn't fully recovered. Upon arrival, I could tell that Terry was not well. She was weak and should not have been released from the hospital. The airline trip had left her severely dehydrated. I had to assist her to my condominium on the second floor. We talked for several hours and she went to the bathroom. Within minutes of entering the bathroom she uttered out, "Roger help me". I rushed to the bathroom to find her head between her knees. I then picked her up and placed her on the bed, where she lay limp. I noticed that her eyes were fixed and staring out in space. I got no pulse. I touched her cornea with my finger with no response. I attempted to use CPR several times with no heart beat or pupillary response. I immediately went to the next room to dial 911, where I became very upset at the operator, as she kept asking a lot of needless questions. I told the operator I thought Terry was dead. Finally, I had to cut the operator short and told her to get HERE NOW, as I needed to get back to continue CPR.

As I returned to the bedroom, I heard a faint moaning in the back room, as Terry had begun to recover. Soon after, the ambulance arrived to take Terry to Naples Hospital #3 for observation. The diagnosis was cardiac arrest from a severe electrolyte imbalance, and a reaction to an oral antifungal agent that had been prescribed prior to leaving Toledo Hospital #1.

One week later, after leaving the hospital, Terry collapsed for a second time, but this time did not lose consciousness. The ambulance arrived but Terry had already recovered, declining return to the hospital for a second time. We had been at a restaurant in attendance with some friends Carol and Hal vacationing from Toledo. While continuing our vacation in Florida over the next two months it became a living hell, as Terry was in and out of Naples

Hospital #3 multiple different times for vomiting and infections. Toward the end of our stay, doctors at Naples #3 suggested the possibility of another intestinal obstruction may have occurred. Finally, I told Terry something is radically wrong, and we need to go back to Toledo Hospital #1. Terry and I packed our suit cases, including all TPN bags and IV sets and drove back to Toledo.

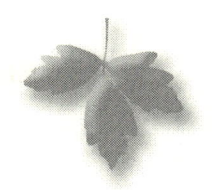

CHAPTER VIII

Upon admittance to Toledo Hospital #1, additional testing was completed revealing an intestinal obstruction was present. While there, Terry arranged for a preliminary exam by one of the Toledo Hospital #1's surgeons. The surgeon informed her, with her history of recent intestinal surgery performed at the Rochester Hospital #2, it could be necessary for her to remain on TPN for life. He suggested she may be unable to eat food in the future. This scared Terry so much she quickly ruled out having surgery performed there.

After that exam, Terry made arrangements to have surgery performed at Cleveland Hospital #4. It took several weeks to get an appointment with the surgeon. When we met the surgeon, we discussed the difficulties Terry had encountered during the post-operative period at Rochester Hospital #2. We discussed the "third spacing" that had occurred, which included a two month stay at the hospital. We informed the surgeon at Cleveland Hospital #4 that doctor's lack of intervention to fluid overload had led to complications that had prolonged her stay. Furthermore, we explained doctor's refusal to use diuretics to control that fluid. We explained this was done on the pretext that diuretics could somehow harm her one kidney. Despite the fact Terry's arms, legs and torso were extremely swollen, doctors still continued to use intravenous fluid that sent her to the intensive care unit on multiple visits. These visits resulted in painful needle taps to her body cavities, both pleural and peritoneal. The surgeon was told of our frustration and my leaving Rochester Hospital #2, and my return to Toledo. Finally, I told the surgeon it was Terry's decision to risk her one kidney, and to be administered diuretics as needed, that eventually allowed her to overcome "third spacing" and leave Rochester Hospital #2. Her decision had resulted in a change of nephrologists and a new plan of action.

Following the Cleveland Hospital #4 surgery, Terry and I were flabbergasted to find out what the surgeon there had discovered. He notified Terry that the obstruction was at the exact spot of reattachment of her bowel from the original surgery at Rochester Hospital #2. The surgeon explained he would not have to remove additional bowel. This was comforting news, in that Terry had feared a new obstruction and further bowel removal. The inability of doctors at the Rochester Hospital #2 to control fluid accumulation inside the abdominal cavity had resulted in suture failure, dehiscence, and the original obstruction to re-obstruct. She had remained obstructed that full year, with the re-obstruction resulting in intermittent vomiting and repeated infections. The only thing saving her life over the last year had been continual use of TPN and the antibiotics.

Several days following Terry's second surgery, I visited her room at the Cleveland Hospital #4. I noticed Terry's difficulty breathing, while attempting to use the commode. Her arms and legs had begun to swell, just as they had at Rochester Hospital #2. The same symptoms were resurfacing. I stepped into the hallway to get a nurse only to see Terry's surgeon. Her surgeon was just completing rounds. I asked that he take a quick look at Terry and reminded him of our discussion preceding her surgery. Fortunately, he listened and immediately prescribed diuretics for several days. Then, Terry had an uneventful recovery. Maintaining her on diuretics made all the difference in the world. She maintained an excellent appetite and was able to continue physical activity. The doctors allowed her access to the commode, and the nurses provided some activity, such as walking.

Upon leaving the hospital, Terry and I were receiving instructions from her surgeon, as to directions to follow when she went home. The surgeon suggested Terry would not have diarrhea any more. I jokingly said something like, "yeah and the world is square" or something like that. Terry had been plagued with persistent diarrhea for over forty years following radiation treatments for ovarian cancer. Despite all the Lomotil and ancillary drugs her stool had always been liquid. The surgeon was insinuating that after forty years his surgery and directions would somehow change her condition of loose stools was ludicrous. The surgeon turned to Terry out of the clear blue sky and said, "just for that, I'm NOT going to issue YOU, meaning Terry, directions". He got up and walked out of the room. It was shocking to me, as I was smiling at the time, and in no way was I insinuating any direct insult to the man. His residents were equally as perplexed as I was. What bothered me the most was he didn't direct his comments toward me, but instead took it out on his patient, Terry. What literature he had for her were NOT dispensed. As a professional I could not imagine such lack of compassion and such an insult to a client! I guess I should still thank him, as his surgery was one of the few bright spots of Terry's hospitalizations, but still it revealed the darkest side of an already dark side of human medicine. For a profession I once envied and respected, I had lost ALL respect. Following his surgery, and with the support of TPN, Terry did quite well for the year of 2015.

From Cleveland Hospital #4, Terry was sent to a rehab clinic that was substandard. Terry wanted to leave the first night she was there. She did not feel safe physically, and the sanitation was unsatisfactory. Her room's flooring was carpet, a surface that could not be easily cleaned, instead of tile or linoleum. In addition, Terry was on an immunosuppressant drug. Imagine sick patients who had diarrhea or vomitus that spilled onto the carpet! The rehab's nutrition provided for a person recovering from malnutrition was extremely poor and that became an issue as well. This rehab facility had been suggested by the Cleveland Hospital #4. Terry asked for an immediate transfer to Toledo, where the facilities were cleaner and where proper nutrition could be provided. I remember Terry had all kinds of difficulties leaving, when requesting transfer to a rehab facility closer in Toledo. What facility wouldn't want the patient to stay longer when a bag of TPN was being charged at $1200 a bag. As I remember, we stayed less than a week. She later filed a report against the rehab clinic for sanitation deficiencies.

It was the spring of 2015, when Terry finally left the rehab clinic. After leaving, Terry's appetite diminished, and she stated she felt nauseated at times. Also, her energy levels had declined. When Terry left the Cleveland Hospital #4, she looked and acted very healthy. I recall the doctors had administered an abundance of corticosteroids, while at the hospital. For years I had thought Terry's vomiting attacks and nausea had some connection to adrenal insufficiency. After all, the radiation treatments had blanketed her entire abdominal area, which over years resulted in loss of her kidney function and a resultant kidney transplant. Terry and I consulted her family physician in Toledo. I explained to her family physician my assessment of why I thought Terry's health had declined after release at Cleveland Hospital #4. While at the hospital, I exclaimed doctors had given Terry heavy doses of corticosteroids. She had shown unusual strength and vitality following surgery. I felt there could be a connection, and that the corticosteroids could now be leaving her system. It could be inferred that since her kidneys had failed from radiation, she might also have suffered adrenal damage. Finally, after years of Terry talking to doctors about adrenal insufficiency, her family physician approved the adrenal drug, Florinef. The improvement was immediate and dramatically improved her remaining life. Terry explained the addition of the drug as a miracle, that for the first time in many years, she experienced appetite for a sustained period of time. This became the longest time for reprieve of Terry's medical problems since her obstruction first surfaced in 2013. Terry continued using TPN throughout 2015, reaching a weight of 94 lbs. by December of that year. She did well that fall, traveling by airplane to Florida and then several weeks later, returning to Toledo.

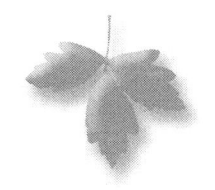

CHAPTER IX

Shortly after returning from our November Florida vacation, Terry received some bad news. As of January 1st, 2016, insurance under Obama Care would no longer pay for TPN administration. Repeated attempts to have TPN reinstituted were continually denied. Beginning in the fall of 2013, Terry's weight had recovered from 78 lbs. to 94 lbs., by the end of 2015. Her weight rapidly dissipated by mid-February 2016 following TPN removal. Terry was hospitalized at Toledo Hospital #1 for malnutrition and multiple infections. With her conditions of short bowel disease and kidney transplant, she was unable to absorb enough food and nutrients resulting in loss of muscle mass, severe malnutrition, and infections from an overwhelmed immune system. Without assistance from TPN, she couldn't absorb enough calories and nutrients orally with her weight plummeting to 82 lbs.. What bowel she still possessed lacked absorptive capacity and food passed undigested. A second problem for Terry was receiving the immune-suppressant drug, tacrolimus, to prevent rejection of her kidney transplant. This was a double-edged sword. She was in a severe state of malnutrition that compromised her immune system, and she was taking immunosuppressant drugs for her kidney transplant, both of which severely retarded her ability to fight off impending infections.

Upon entry to Toledo Hospital #1, intravenous TPN therapy was reinstituted. Multiple antibiotics were administered to fight off the infections that had begun to overwhelm her. I was in Florida when Terry notified me that she had been hospitalized. I suggested she contact our political representative in Bowling Green, to see if he could alter Medicare's decision to reinstitute TPN. Within seventy-two hours, his office had Medicare's approval for Terry to receive TPN for life. Unfortunately, that decision came too little too late, as the damage had already been done. She never fully recovered from those infections, as they continued to plague her throughout 2016. Upon leaving the hospital in the spring of 2016, Terry continued the use of TPN, but soon developed an abscess of the cervical spine and infections involving both her retinas. I returned from Florida to assist her during that time. The antibiotic used to control her infections, Daptomycin, resulted in severe anorexia, weight loss, and fluid accumulation. For a while she had to briefly discontinue this therapy, due to the severe side effects from the drug. Terry's circumstances, with short bowel disease and kidney transplant, spared her few oral drug offerings due to the side effects that would often accompany her conditions, as diarrhea and vomiting. Also, some oral drugs would be poorly absorbed.

By the fall of 2016, the Toledo Hospital #1 had resolved most of Terry's medical issues, and she was driving her car again, had gained weight, and decided to accompany me back to Florida for a short vacation. Terry had four cats which she loved and could not stay away from for a long period of time. She planned to stay two weeks in Naples, Florida, and return to Toledo by airplane. We packed our suit cases and left for Florida on 11/15/2016. The drive down was uneventful. Terry made arrangements for the local TPN distributors in Tampa, Florida, to deliver the TPN to Naples.

Upon arrival in Florida, she received confirmation for approval of the drug, Gattex, recently approved by the FDA to improve short bowel disease absorption. The drug increased elongation of the intestinal villus as well as its absorptive capacity, giving new hopes for people receiving TPN. The drug had recent approval in

Europe, two years earlier, and the United States recently gained approval as well. Terry had sought approval for nearly a year, with acceptance and rejection on several occasions. One rejection was that she had cancer, even though she had been rendered ovarian cancer free for some forty plus years. For a patient with active cancer it was a contraindication to receive the drug, Gattex. Terry and I believed Medicare and the insurance companies were trying to delay or prevent access to her care. The reason for approval delay was MONEY! The cost of a bag of TPN was $1200 a bag and most patients were dispensed from five to seven bags a week. The drug, Gattex, listed price was $300,000 annually. Finally, after many delays, the drug representative from Shire intervened and assured the opposition Terry did not currently have cancer. Shire was the company responsible for Gattex distribution here in the United States. The drug was to arrive in Naples within one week, and I was to assist Terry in administering the drug, while she was vacationing. Subcutaneous was the route for administration. Oral improvement of absorption of nutrients for people who had short bowel disease had been demonstrated. As patients received the drug for an interval of time, which could vary from individual to individual, they needed less maintenance of TPN. Many patients were able to reduce the total number of bags of TPN weekly, but some patients had supposedly been completely weaned from TPN. Patients demonstrated weight gain and increased muscle mass. Overall patients appeared healthier with increased vitality resulting in reduction in overall morbidity.

Then everything changed. Only days after arriving in Florida, Terry awakened unable to ambulate. Sensory sensation was present, but she suffered severe motor deficits and could no longer walk. We were in a quandary as what to do. All plans made were immediately abandoned, including the use of the drug, Gattex. We decided, since we had been satisfied with treatment in Toledo earlier, it was necessary for us to turn around ten days after our arrival in Florida and drive all the way back to Toledo. An airplane was considered, but we disbanded that idea with Terry's circumstance with paresis plus the additional short bowel disease and diarrhea. Therefore, we quickly repacked our suitcases, and began our quest back to Toledo Hospital #1 for consultation. Unfortunately, I lived on the second floor of my condominium. First, it was necessary to close out all utilities and ancillary services that had been recently initiated. Then, I loaded up all Terry's TPN fluids, intravenous sets and pole, and all our luggage. My next project was to safely carry Terry down two flights of stairs. Finally, I grabbed my companion "snooter' and her dog food, and off we went.

Once in the car, Terry and I both became keenly aware of an additional obstacle, most notable was Terry's short bowel problems and paresis. I needed to figure out a method to deal with her loose stools. It didn't help that she was virtually paralyzed. After much thought, I decided on a bed pan that I could slip under her, when she found it necessary to relieve herself. As we began the trek back to Toledo, I thought it would never end. Terry decided against eating anything, since that would have made our travel much more time consuming. We made the trip back in two days, stopping at a motel just long enough to administer her TPN.

When we arrived at Toledo Hospital #1, we went directly to the emergency room, as this hospital had always been her hospital of choice. I went to the waiting room, as there were lots of sick patients. Upon admittance, Terry was placed in an emergency room waiting several hours for tests to be performed. When I returned, I was disillusioned at the doctor's diagnosis, and how Terry was to be handled. Terry had recently been hospitalized at this same institution several times in early winter and again in late spring 2016. We had just traveled twelve hundred miles to go to Toledo Hospital #1's emergency room and could have just as easily stopped at one of many hospitals along the way, only to be turned away by the emergency physician stating that Terry's condition of paresis did NOT warrant hospitalization.

The physician's diagnosis was a urinary tract infection. Furthermore, the doctor was SENDING HER HOME with antibiotics! I was shocked! What about Terry's leg paresis and her inability to walk I inquired? What testing of her legs have you completed? Have you examined her legs at all? I explained I was a veterinarian, and his diagnosis of a urinary tract infection, as a cause of her paresis, did not even remotely seem plausible. He then reaffirmed that paresis was NOT a reason to hospitalize a patient sent to an emergency room. I asked him to check Terry's records, as she had been a recent patient there. It did no good. He was adamant that Terry was NOT going to be admitted to the hospital. It made absolutely no sense that emergency personnel are trained to take extreme caution when handling spinal trauma cases, yet hospitalization wasn't necessary for a patient exhibiting paresis! Finally, I informed the doctor unless he did tests for causes of paresis, he would have to "just keep her" and I left quite upset.

Three hours later, the hospital called stating neurological tests had been completed, but results would not be available until the next day. The nurse informed me Terry wanted to go home. I had driven from Florida, arriving at their hospital emergency room at four pm, and now seven hours later, at eleven pm, I was going back to the hospital for the second time. Terry and I finally got home at eleven-thirty that night. I began to unpack our bags, dreary from the long trip from Florida. Terry began her antibiotics immediately that night.

Throughout the next day, I knew something just wasn't right with Terry. I called a friend of hers, Sue, to come to the house to visit Terry. I informed Sue of the incident that happened at Toledo Hospital #1 the night before. When Sue arrived, it was evening and time for Terry to program her TPN. Sue and I went to the bedroom, while Terry attempted to program her TPN. She became confused as to how to accomplish it. At that point I told Sue, Terry needs to go back to the hospital. Terry had always been sharp mentally. There was something seriously wrong. I was unsure what hospital to admit her, due to the situation that developed at Toledo Hospital #1 the night before. Finally, I called another of Terry's friends, Susan, who had assisted Terry while at the Rochester Hospital #2. Susan suggested that I call an ambulance, as the hospital she would be sent would be forced to accept her. I decided it would be best to send Terry by ambulance back to Toledo Hospital #1. She was hospitalized there on 11/29/2016.

While there, she was placed on intravenous fluids and treated with antibiotics for sepsis, but days into her treatment, the hospital was doing nothing to address her paresis. I visited her daily, but the doctors failed to arrive at a consensus, as to the cause of her paresis. Finally, after Terry's continued insistence to have diagnostic work done on her paresis, the work was finally completed but results were still not forth coming.

Then on December 6th, I arrived at the hospital at nine am to find Terry had vomited all night. Apparently, the nurses had neglected to give her reflux medication she relied upon. She appeared quite dehydrated, and the doctors had not yet initiated any replacement fluid therapy. I was visibly upset, as Terry's condition appeared to be worsening. She had been there a week, and doctors still had not approached her paresis. There was no goal in sight. Terry and I discussed the situation that had been unfolding at Toledo Hospital #1, as to the lack of concern on admittance at the emergency room. Now, there appeared to be lack of concern for her health after being admitted. She had been a patient there for years. We decided her surgery one year earlier at Cleveland Hospital #4 had been successful, so we would return there. On the very morning we made the decision to go to Cleveland Hospital #4, the doctors at Toledo Hospital #1 released information that Terry had a spinal abscess located in the lumbar spine. The doctors proclaimed it was a surgery their surgeons could easily perform there at Toledo Hospital #1. I do not understand why this information had not been released earlier.

Once we decided to go to Cleveland Hospital #4, we experienced unexpected pressure to remain at Toledo Hospital #1. Multiple doctors were sent to Terry's room in an attempt to sway her decision to stay at Toledo Hospital #1 for treatment. They kept asking Terry over and over again whether she wanted to remain at Toledo Hospital #1. She continued to tell them she had made the decision to leave for Cleveland Hospital #4. They accused me, as her power of attorney, of attempting to sway her opinion. The constant barrage of doctors was very upsetting, as Terry was already dealing with physical and mental issues about her condition. Their pressure was so intense that shouting arguments ensued, and a security guard was called. I had visited Terry at nine am, argued till eleven am, and now it was 5 pm that evening, when we finally returned home. Terry and I picked up Snooter, reshuffled our needed clothes and medication, to continue our trek onward toward Cleveland.

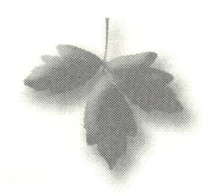

CHAPTER X

We arrived at the Cleveland Hospital #4 emergency room at ten pm on 12/06/16. Two hours later, Terry was moved to an examination room at the emergency clinic. I stayed with her at the room leaving necessary information about myself, as name, phone number, and that I would be staying at the Red Roof Inn just outside of Cleveland. Because I had my dog Snooter in my presence, I left for the Red Roof Inn.

The next morning, I visited Terry at nine am at the Cleveland Hospital #4. She was in a recovery room and informed me that at two am that morning, or within two hours of me leaving for the motel, a surgeon had completed emergency surgery on the spinal abscess. Terry was mentally alert, and her recovery appeared excellent. She was elated that she again had the ability to use her legs. She even, while lying on her back, lifted her legs and moved her toes vigorously. She was doing so well, that an hour later, I kissed her good bye, and I returned to Toledo to complete long overdue paper work. The news suggested a large snow storm was due to move into the area shortly. I told Terry I would stay in touch with her by cell phone, and that I would return to pick her up in several days. Soon after I left, Terry called a friend of hers, Debbie, notifying Debbie the surgery was a success and that she could use her legs again. Terry informed Debbie she expected to leave the hospital in three to five days for a rehab site. Later, her medical report from the surgeon substantiated that same time frame.

On 12/07/16, that same night, as I returned to Toledo the storm hit. The storm was quite severe, closing roads for several days making travel almost impossible. I called the nurses responsible for Terry's care daily. I was unable to contact Terry on the cell phone and, when I asked the nurse if I could talk to her, Terry was always unavailable, with some nurse, doctor, or other medical personnel in attendance. Then, I was asked to call back. Terry's nurses suggested she was doing fine. On 12/10/16 when I talked to her nurse, she informed me Terry had torn her Foley catheter out of her bladder and had done some bleeding. I asked how serious it was, and whether despite all the bad weather, I should attempt to go to Cleveland. The nurse assured me that the doctors had everything under control. When I contacted Terry's nurse the next day, she continued to insist Terry was fine. I asked the nurse why Terry had not called me on her cell phone. She replied Terry had not charged her cell phone. I asked the nurse to please charge her cell phone for her. That never happened! I began to become concerned.

On 12/14/2016 the roads cleared, and I notified Terry's hospital nurse I was coming to Cleveland that morning to visit her. Upon receiving my call, the nurse handed the phone to a doctor, who said Terry may be sent to a nursing home. I asked why I hadn't been informed of her declining condition, as when I left she appeared normal. I told him all pertinent information had been left with their hospital personnel to contact me. He tried to exclaim it away they had called the wrong phone number. Upon arrival at Terry's room at Cleveland Hospital #4, I was greeted by the doctor, I had previously talked to, and a nurse. I couldn't believe the difference in Terry's condition from when I left her. Her head was slumped over, and she was unaware of my presence. Her arms, legs, and torso were practically unrecognizable, laden with fluid two to three times normal. I looked up to see an intravenous bag dangling from an IV stand still dripping fluid into her vein. Where had I seen this picture before? Could it have been at Rochester #2? In addition, instead of a commode by her bedside, these doctors had also inserted a rectal hose to remove Terry's feces.

In no uncertain words, I immediately complained to the doctor and nurse that the fluids were the problem. I said, "you're drowning her in fluids". As her power of attorney, I immediately informed hospital personnel to remove all fluids, other than blood and antibiotics. I requested they institute use of a diuretic, such as Lasix, which doctors refused. These doctors at Cleveland Hospital #4 were quoting the same old adage Rochester Hospital #2 had. They suggested diuretics would somehow compromise her kidney transplant! My reply was you are compromising her life! I asked doctors to please check Terry's Cleveland Hospital #4 records for 2014. Just one year earlier, the surgeon and doctors at that same facility had instituted diuretics controlling her "third spacing" for a smooth recovery. They REFUSED to check Terry's prior medical records. Instead, doctors found it more important for hospital personnel to check the validity of my claim, that I was her power of attorney.

In 2014, I had submitted and had approval for all necessary documents for Terry's re-obstruction surgery. Now doctors proclaimed my power of attorney, that I had submitted in 2014, lacked one page, the last page, for notarization. Without that final page, doctors threatened to remove my power of attorney. Under duress, I returned to Toledo on a Sunday to obtain an affidavit proving my assertion that I was, in fact, her power of attorney. While there, I had problems making contact with her original attorney, as his office was closed. Terry's documents had been filed some five years earlier. The attorney's recorder at his office indicated he would be unavailable for an indeterminate time due to illness. In a panic, I attempted to contact his residence by cell phone. Hours later, I was able to make contact at his residence, where he was recovering from cancer treatments. Due to the circumstances I found myself in, he was nice enough to return to his office and provide an affidavit.

That same night, after obtaining the affidavit, I returned to Cleveland Hospital #4 unsure of my course of action. What I was certain of, was I wasn't going to continue to allow them to drown Terry in fluid! I reasoned she was unable to accept solid food, but yogurt she could swallow and ice chips would add fluid if she needed it. I further reasoned that her one kidney would gradually remove excess fluid, and any additional fluid would gradually return to her circulatory system by homeostasis. So, from 12/14/2016 until 12/22/2016, Terry's fluid gradually receded, readjusted and redistributed throughout her body, since no intravenous therapy had been given. She improved markedly demonstrating renewed strength and vitality. She went from being near comatose to being able to hold her head erect and readily accepted yogurt and ice chips. I reasoned she could soon begin to eat solid foods, which was so necessary to recover from her "third spacing".

Then, on 12/22/2016, a TPN doctor came to our room insisting he needed to begin TPN, otherwise Terry risk dying from malnutrition. I reluctantly agreed ONLY if he would agree NOT to give Terry so much fluid, as to return her to her original state. He was to reduce not only the total amount of fluid, but the flow rate as well. He shrugged his shoulders as to agree. Within 36 hours, the TPN doctors had administered even more fluid, as she was worse than when I arrived on 12/14/2016, the day I used my power of attorney to stop all fluids. The TPN doctors had infused so much fluid her body weight mushroomed from 122 lbs. on 12/22/2016, when they were given permission to resume TPN, to 143 lbs. on 12/24/2016 when I discontinued TPN for the second time.

Her body weight upon admission was only 88 lbs.. From admission three weeks earlier, the doctors had added 55 lbs. of fluid to a patient that had only one kidney. Her normal weight over the last 3 years was in a range of 88 lbs. to 94 lbs.. I will forever blame myself for allowing doctors to reinstitute fluids! You want to trust hospital personnel! Sadly, there can be NO TRUST! I was extremely angry that all the improvement Terry had shown was gone. The doctors had lied to me! They had used no common sense. Again, I reiterated to the doctors what I had stated before, that their own hospital, Cleveland Hospital #4, had used diuretics to successfully control her third spacing just one year earlier. An argument ensued that was so heated a security guard was called. Cleveland Hospital #4 security threatened to have me removed from the hospital premises. Rather than removal, I found it necessary to try to fight for Terry's life. I talked to the ombudsman which was a complete waste of time. I decided to return to what had served me well in the past, which was yogurt and ice chips.

After this second "third spacing" event at Cleveland Hospital #4. I was much more worried, as Terry, even though able to swallow, exhibited more lassitude and semi-conscious behavior than when I arrived on 12/14/2016. From that morning, of December 24th, Terry was still attempting to consume ice chips and yogurt but not as aggressively as before. Then at four pm Christmas Eve, one of the doctors, who witnessed Terry's earlier recovery, was accomplishing rounds. I informed him of what had happened to Terry and asked his advice. He seemed surprised at her condition, as he had watched her gradual improvement. When asked about Lasix, he said there was nothing he could do. He suggested I continue as before, as he had seen the progress she had made in the past. Soon after the doctor left his shift, as I continued the use of ice chips and yogurt, Terry suddenly began exhibiting intermittent hand contractures later identified as myoclonic. She reached to the ceiling and then slowly relaxed her hands to return to the original position. These hand contractures would last for several minutes, disappear for half an hour, and then would reoccur. I was unsure of these symptoms, so I called the nurse. She knew absolutely nothing.

As Christmas Eve approached ten pm, Terry's symptoms increased. Not only was she experiencing hand contractures, but by midnight, muscle spasms had engaged her esophagus and spirally wound its way from the cervical region dorsally up her mouth. As a veterinarian small animal practitioner for over 40 years I had never seen anything quite like this in animals. No longer could I administer Terry anything orally, less I risk foreign body pneumonia. I called the nurse requesting she summon the on-call physician as soon as possible. It took the attending doctor two hours to arrive at Terry's room, as it now was two am Christmas Day. The on-call doctor could not identify Terry's symptoms. I explicitly asked the doctor if it could be an epileptic event but she replied, "no". She suggested that I turn the lights out and allow Terry to go to sleep She insinuated Terry's symptoms would just go away. I had requested Gatorade earlier in the evening which Terry had ingested, thinking the spasms could be related to electrolyte imbalances. As the night drifted into the early morning hours of Christmas Day, her hand contractures and esophageal spasms seemed to dissipate. At four am, I thought it safe to leave, so I summoned the nurse and asked that she keep a close eye on Terry. She assured me that she would.

The next morning, I arrived at Terry's room about ten am, and was told Terry had been moved to a different ward. Hospital personnel described it as the coronary unit. When I arrived at that room, I was shocked. Terry had been intubated on a respirator and was lying on a mobile bed. She was whisked away for additional testing. When she returned, she could no longer recognize me. In viewing her, I was fearful she had sustained brain damage, as earlier symptoms appeared to me to be neurological. The left side of her neck was notably swollen to the size of two golf balls, where the esophageal spasms had originated. The esophageal muscle had hypertrophied. This occurrence could only have been explained by violent and sustained muscular contractions-extreme seizure activity. Left uncontrolled seizures can result in permanent brain damage. Since it was early Christmas Day, it is quite possible hospital personnel failed to closely monitor Terry.

It is my belief when Terry's symptoms first became apparent, and neither the doctor nor the nurse could identify her problem, she should have been sent immediately to an intensive care unit for twenty-four-hour observation. This is especially true, since it was during the period of Christmas Eve and Christmas Day. Earlier neurological symptoms were a harbinger of what was to follow-an epileptic event. The timing couldn't have been worse. She only remained at the coronary unit for a brief time, and doctors decided to relocate her to the nephrology unit. I asked myself. How could her condition get so out of control? I began to have serious doubts of Terry ever recovering and little information had been offered.

Terry looked absolutely horrible, as her arms and legs were still extremely swollen from the volume of fluid TPN doctors had administered. Upon admission, Terry originally had two small bed sores, but after doctors had confined her to the rectal hose, it created bed sores more expansive and added new ones. Prior to restarting TPN administration on 12/22/2016, her creatinine, a kidney function test, was 1.88, but after the seizure event jumped quickly to 2.3. Over the next six days her creatinine jumped to 3.7, as her kidney began to fail. Cleveland Hospital #4's version of Terry's event, was a hypotensive, anaphylactic reaction due to a blood transfusion. Questions immediately arose, as no hospital personnel mentioned anything about any blood transfusion being necessary. In the past, doctors had always requested prior approval. I don't believe their final version of events.

I had questions concerning Terry's brain function, but the doctors would not provide any information. Also, I inquired if they had completed an encephalogram, but again answers were not forthcoming. I went to Toledo to bring Terry's sister-in-law, Kathy, to Cleveland to visit Terry the day after her event. Kathy immediately questioned the enlargement on the left side of Terry's neck. I informed Kathy it was the exact site Terry had experienced esophageal spasms the night preceding her serious event.

While at Cleveland Hospital #4, Kathy and I discussed Terry's condition. The important decision to return Terry to Toledo was made, as her kidney function continued to decline and dialysis hadn't been considered. Arrangements for her return were not made easily as Cleveland Hospital #4 was in charge. The first thing they informed me was that insurance would not cover Terry's transfer to Toledo Hospital #5 from the Cleveland Hospital #4 because both hospitals were the same level of care. Therefore, insurance would not cover the $1500 expense to transfer Terry back to Toledo. I informed the hospital I didn't care what the expense. I just wanted her out of Cleveland Hospital #4! Arrangements were made for an ambulance service in Toledo to drive to Cleveland Hospital #4, receive Terry, and return her to Toledo. On 1/02/17, as the ambulance arrived at Cleveland Hospital #4, doctors upon removal of the rectal hose from Terry, experienced gushing of blood from her rectum. As a result, a Cleveland Hospital #4 doctor informed me while in Toledo, that Terry needed a blood transfusion. The doctor wanted to keep Terry overnight to give the blood transfusion at their hospital. I informed the doctor to begin the blood transfusion but send Terry by ambulance directly to Toledo Hospital #5, that Cleveland Hospital #4 had done ENOUGH!

Upon arrival at Toledo Hospital #5, Terry was given a bed. Myself and Terry's sister-in-law, Kathy, were awaiting her arrival. As we visited, Terry appeared very much at ease. Though unable to talk or move her eyes much, I could sense her relief she was back in Toledo. The rooms were much bigger and the light abundant, unlike the dismal rooms provided at the Cleveland Hospital #4. The Toledo Hospital #5 doctors reviewed Terry's medical reports and did a preliminary examination. They revealed what I had expected, that the chances of her recovery were remote. Despite the extremely poor prognosis, not revealed at Cleveland Hospital #4, we decided to move forward with dialysis at Toledo Hospital #5. The first treatment there was unsuccessful. The doctors suggested possibly better success at Toledo Hospital #1, as they had newer, more advanced equipment. We then transported Terry back to Toledo Hospital #1 for additional dialysis treatments, in the hopes her kidney function could change her overall condition.

From 1/02/2017 until 1/09/2017, Terry's condition deteriorated further, as all of her vital organs began to fail. It became apparent that her condition involved her brain, something that doctors at Cleveland Hospital #4 had not revealed to me. Her blood pressure began dropping precipitously. The doctors increased her blood pressure medications from one drug to three just to keep her alive. Her distal extremities began to turn from pink to blue-black. The time Terry and I had once talked about, but never expected, removing her from life support was near. Terry's friend, Sue, joined Kathy and myself in the hospital waiting room. We talked for several hours about her condition, then proceeded to her room to wish Terry our last farewell. I signed the necessary documents to remove her from life support. We then left. Minutes after leaving I received the message that the love of my life, Terry had passed away.

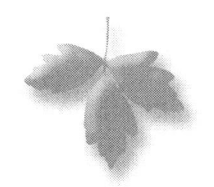

CHAPTER XI

After her death, I was named executor, but I wanted to return to Florida just to get away. Terry's sister-in-law assisted in contacting the funeral home concerning Terry's cremation. Terry was a very private person, not wanting a funeral viewing or reception. She wanted her cremains be given to Rudy, her ex-husband, and myself, her companion for nearly thirty years. She wanted her ashes disbursed on the beaches in Hawaii, where Rudy now lives, and the beaches of Naples, Florida, where I reside. She loved Naples, Florida, but was never able to fully enjoy the area due to the illnesses that would always seem to interrupt her, while we were vacationing. I designated her attorney to assume the obligation of taking care of her estate as executor. For the next month and a half, I assisted him in Toledo.

One of the most difficult chores was to find homes for her four cats. I was allergic to cats and had severe asthma, when around them for any period of time. Therefore, my caring for her cats was out of the question. Terry's wishes for her cats had been scribbled onto a piece of paper several weeks before we left for our last Florida vacation in the fall of 2016. Terry had written she wanted her cats all euthanatized, but at the end of her statement, she placed a big question mark. She knew it would be difficult to place all four cats at the same home, due to the one cat's advancing age. She preferred the cats all remain together. In the end, I felt that big question mark meant Terry did NOT want her cats put to sleep, if other arrangements could be made. The cat's names were Gracie, Pea Pod, Harvey, and String Bean. The most social was Gracie, as she had lots of friends outside. One of Terry's next-door neighbors had rescued Gracie from an abandoned house several years earlier, and had informed Terry, if Gracie ever needed a home the neighbor would take her. The other three cats became a problem, especially Harvey the fourteen year-year old. After a month of attempting to find homes for the remaining three cats, Kathy, Terry's sister-in-law, was forced to send them to the local Humane Society. Kathy requested all three cats occupy the same home if possible. When I returned to Toledo in mid-May 2017, the first place I stopped was the local Humane Society. All three cats had found homes, hopefully with the same owner.

Upon returning to Florida in February of 2016, I embarked on assembling information on what had gone horribly wrong. I knew something very sinister must have occurred for Terry's health to spiral out of control in one week. The fact that Cleveland Hospital #4 did not contact me during that week was very unsettling. While in Florida, I requested Terry's attorney retrieve Terry's medical reports from Cleveland Hospital #4. I began the painstaking job of deciphering what was important and what was not, as Cleveland Hospital #4 had over seven hundred pages in her medical reports. It took me over one month to read and understand them. The fact I was a veterinarian made me familiar with most of the medical drugs, supplies, and medical jargon. Still, seven hundred pages were a lot of pages to visualize. In addition to deciding what facts were important, I also needed to build a timeline for events that transpired. Slowly, I began to assimilate what I thought was a reasonable explanation for what had gone wrong.

The most alarming thing was twenty-four hours after I returned to Toledo, Terry immediately began to experience delirium. The Cleveland Hospital #4 made no attempt to contact me, despite the fact I left all pertinent information as my name, address, phone number, and the motel, where I would be staying. When I asked the doctor, upon returning to the hospital, why I hadn't been alerted to her declining condition, he stated he called the wrong phone number. Terry's medical reports made it obvious that hospital personnel did not want me to know. I had contact with Terry's nurses daily, and the nurses could have relayed any important information from doctors concerning Terry's declining health. As for the nurses, they relayed no negative medical information, leading me to believe that Terry had been recovering. One of Terry's nurses stated the reason Terry had not called me on her cell phone was she hadn't charged her cell phone, now appear less than truthful. Terry's medical reports indicate Terry had been experiencing delirium from the first day after recovery following her surgery and wouldn't have been capable of charging her cell phone, much less make a phone call!

At the recovery room, Terry's surgeon had suggested a three to five-day hospitalization, followed by release to a rehab clinic. I feel it unlikely the surgeon revisited Terry again, as he was an emergency surgeon, unlikely to follow up on individual cases. Following a short stay at the recovery room, Terry had been transferred to a different room. Then, doctors administered by injections the drugs, Dilaudid and Morphine, for pain, and oral Trazadone for sleep. Within twenty-four hours of initiation of these drugs, Terry began to exhibit symptoms of delirium. Due to the suddenness of her change in condition, she apparently had a reaction to the drug, Dilaudid, or the combination of drugs, resulting in her delirium. Doctors were apparently unable to identify the cause for her delirium. Dilaudid is a common drug used in many hospital settings. Delirium is just one of the side effects of Dilaudid. In fact, Dilaudid has special warnings for patients with impaired kidney function, such as a kidney transplant as Terry. Despite removal of Dilaudid from the patient, sometimes the drug's side effects can persist for days. It was noted that after two doses of Dilaudid, the doctors reduced Terry's Dilaudid dose by half, but then continued the drugs Dilaudid and Trazadone for three additional days. These drugs should have been removed completely!

Following drug administration, Terry began to experience delirium that resulted in bowel incontinence, to which doctors elected to apply a rectal hose for removal of any fecal material. Rather than have nurses assist Terry through her recovery with a commode, doctors placed her in confinement with a RECTAL HOSE, in which it would have been nearly IMPOSSIBLE to give her any necessary physical therapy. She was malnourished and weak following surgery. Doctors chose convenience and sanitation with little regard to patient recovery! I suggest that doctors responsible for setting this in motion should have to spend ONE day confined to a rectal hose. If this situation created such an inconvenience, didn't Cleveland Hospital #4 possess a quarantine room?

In past hospital settings, Terry had always had access to a commode, and been assisted by nurses if necessary. In sifting through Terry's medical reports, the rectal hose had been mentioned only once, identified as FMS, probably fecal management system. No mention of when, why, and who was responsible for this heinous act was present in her medical reports. You could tell the hospital did not wish to publicize THIS DEVICE. Terry, as a former health care provider and a patient, the subject of a rectal hose never had been discussed. Despite multiple hospital settings during the last three years, the use of a rectal hose was neither implemented nor discussed.

Which leads me to ask the important question, as to what RIGHT did Cleveland Hospital #4, or any hospital for that matter, have to impose a RECTAL HOSE on a patient without either family approval or power of attorney permission? Do doctors or hospitals have, at their discretion, the right to administer or dispense ANY medical device or instrument they feel appropriate on an unsuspecting patient, especially one suffering from delirium? How demeaning! How life threatening!

While discussing this subject, there are additional issues that I find repulsive. The rectal hose is being placed in an environment that contains potentially lethal bacteria. Terry was receiving immunosuppressant drugs to prevent rejection of her kidney transplant, which would have made her much more vulnerable to any infections. Any irritation or mucosal tear would leave her in a precarious situation. This is why gastrointestinal surgeons are constantly operating on patients for such problems, as diverticulitis, appendicitis, etc.. A rectal hose is NOT like a Foley catheter, whereby the device is introduced into most often a sterile environment, certainly unlike the bowel, a bacterial cesspool.

Even more appalling was in last two years, Terry had experienced two bowel surgeries in the prior two years. The first bowel surgery in 2013 at Rochester Hospital #2 was for an obstruction, but also resulted in much of her bowel being removed resulting in the condition termed short bowel disease. The second bowel surgery in 2014 had been completed at Cleveland Hospital #4 the following year. Why would a doctor apply a rectal hose to such a patient?

In addition, medical reports submitted from other hospitals to Cleveland Hospital #4 contained information concerning her chronic, debilitating radiation disease. Radiation exposure results in ever-lasting capillary fragility, whereby tissues that are damaged easily, refuse to clot, and bleed continuously. Some three weeks after the rectal hose had been imposed, its removal resulted in an intestinal ulceration, such as to cause gushing of blood requiring a blood transfusion. The imposition of the rectal hose resulted in severe intestinal bleeding from damaged tissues. Quite possibly, Terry had been seeping blood soon after its installation, as she received several blood transfusions during her tenure at Cleveland Hospital #4.

Another problem that worsened as a result of the rectal hose were decubital sores, small upon admission to Cleveland Hospital #4, but dramatically expanded, and new sores were created as a result of her confinement and inability to reposition and rotate herself. This confinement made it impossible for Cleveland Hospital #4 to administer physical therapy. During her entire stay at Cleveland Hospital #4, not ONCE did I see any nurse attempt to walk Terry. For nearly a month, Terry's entire stay at Cleveland Hospital #4, she had been confined to a rectal hose. Terry should have been the LEAST LIKELY person to be subjected to a rectal hose. The rectal hose should be BANNED!

Then on 12/10/2016, I called Terry's nurse who stated Terry had torn her Foley catheter from her bladder and bleeding had occurred. When asked how serious her condition was, the nurse remarked doctors had stopped the bleeding and the situation was under control. I asked if I should return to Cleveland Hospital #4 despite the inclement weather, as many roads were closed. She insisted it wasn't necessary. Upon review of Terry's medical reports that was untrue, as bleeding continued for days. Eventually, on 12/18/2016, an additional surgery, cauterization of bleeding capillaries in the bladder, was completed. Blood transfusions followed. Despite cauterization continual bladder capillary seepage continued for weeks, as blood was present in her urine even after she was returned to Toledo weeks later. Blood transfusions resulting from the rectal hose and Foley catheter were complications driven by BAD doctor decisions. These complications had nothing to do with her prior admission for a relatively benign spinal abscess surgical procedure. This was negligence on the part of hospital personnel, as doctors were aware of Terry's radiation disease.

In further review of Terry's medical reports, Terry's delirium was apparent the day after surgical recovery on 12/08/2016. At this time doctors were aware of medical hardware they had applied to Terry, the Foley catheter and the rectal hose. Also, they most certainly should have been aware of her radiation disease. Why then had medical restraints not been applied? Patients suffering from delirium can cause serious self-inflicted bodily injury to themselves, if not properly restrained or monitored, which is exactly what happened. This is especially true since she had radiation disease and, her tissues when damaged would be expected to bleed continuously. Through her hospital stay she suffered multiple blood transfusions due to her self-inflicted injury, not due to her original spinal abscess surgery.

Then, questions arise as to, was her delirium the cause of her tearing her Foley catheter from her bladder or, more plausible, did Terry find herself in a fearful circumstance, desperately attempting to free herself from confinement to the rectal hose and Foley catheter? Knowing Terry, the second possibility sounds most likely! She had already experienced two months of hell several years earlier at Rochester Hospital #2 in 2013. This was far worse due to her confinement, and her lack of ability to move about. You as a patient in a strange environment, with strange people you don't know, being given drugs that immobilize not only your mind but your physical as well, what would you do? The natural inclination would be to attempt to free yourself!

What is most concerning being why doctors and nurses never thought about the predicament their patient found herself? Further review of Terry's medical records revealed that, upon admission on 12/07/2016, her body weight was 88 lbs.. Her body weight within a week rapidly escalated to 122 lbs. on 12/14/2016, when I had returned to Cleveland Hospital #4. This is also the date doctors suggested Terry might be sent to a nursing home. Her arms and legs were severely swollen with fluid, and she was unable to communicate with me. I asked hospital personnel, as her power of attorney, to discontinue all TPN and fluids, except blood and antibiotics. Then on 12/22/2016, the TPN was reinstituted for 36 hours when TPN doctors, for a second time, flooded her with intravenous fluid.

By 12/23/2016 and 12/24/2016, her recorded weight was 143 lbs.. I requested removal of fluids again on 12/23/2016. So, what was originally an 88 lb. malnourished surgical patient upon hospital admittance, had blossomed into a 143 lb. fluid, laden human being, as to become nearly unrecognizable

The "third spacing" fluid accumulation diminished Terry's appetite and destroyed her ability to exercise. Additionally, the excess fluid in her pleural and peritoneal cavities suppressed function of valuable organs and compressed blood vessels. Also, because she had only one functional kidney, the fluid compromised it as well. Multiple attempts to get doctors at Cleveland Hospital #4 to administer diuretics on 12/23/2016 were denied, just as they had been on 12/14/2016. These denials were despite, that in 2014, Cleveland Hospital #4's own surgeon had used diuretics on an, as needed basis to control and manage a similar "third spacing" event. She had a smooth recovery there lasting only one week. I asked doctors to check past hospital records, but they refused. Nurses notes attest to my plea! Thus, the total amount of fluid since admittance was an astonishing 55 lbs. or 60% of her original body weight. Over the last three years, Terry's weight had been in a range of between 88 lbs. and 94 lbs.. Amazingly, despite the huge quantity of fluid her one kidney attempted to process, her kidney function, although elevated, was still in an acceptable mode until after 12/25/2016 when she suffered the seizure.

Following the seizure, she suffered brain damage, resulting in a dramatic lowering of her blood pressure. Over the next ten days, she suffered multiple organ failure and was placed on life support. The emergency physician at Cleveland Hospital #4 lacked the competency to understand Terry's symptoms and did NOT send Terry to a twenty-four-hour intensive care unit on Christmas Day costing her life. The emergency physician also did not file a report, or if filed, was deleted from Terry's medical reports. Terry's medical report issued by Cleveland Hospital #4 was edited as a hypotensive, anaphylactic reaction due to a blood transfusion, rather than an epileptic event. Her medical reports issued other possible explanations for her event making definitive causes questionable.

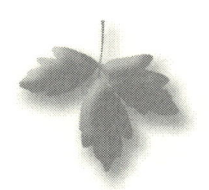

CHAPTER XII

After I had completed all 700 pages of Terry's medical reports, I was sure that some of the various agencies would listen to my complaints, since it involved a death and an individual like myself connected to the medical community. What a quagmire! In March of 2017, I filed complaints with the Joint Commission, Medicare, and the State Medical Board. It had been six months, and I had received NO contact from any of the above agencies. So, I enlisted an attorney friend to send a letter to the State Medical Board. On the very day he sent his letter, I received an email from the State Medical Board informing me there was not enough evidence to pursue her case and that the case was CLOSED. I followed up their email with a phone call. The State Medical Board again stated the case remained closed, unless other additional charges of malpractice from other sources came forward. The materials I had submitted would remain on file for two years. Interestingly, the State Medical Board seemed more interested in prosecuting medical professionals for drug infractions rather than pursuing cases concerned with patient care.

Then, there is the Joint Commission whose responsibilities are to make suggestions on improving patient care and sanitation. The Joint Commission is financially supported by the very hospitals that accredit them. That's like the fox guarding the hen's coop! They make no determinations concerning doctor malpractice. Then, I began to realize something really terrifying. There are few controls in human medicine. Upon showing Terry's medical reports to an attorney friend of mine he exclaimed, "if that had been my wife, I wouldn't have known and probably would have shaken the doctor's hands and thanked them for trying their best".

There have been few reports about the number of deaths due to medical mistakes in the United States. One report suggests that hospital and medical mistakes are the third leading cause of death behind heart disease and cancer. I believe that author to be correct, but to prove it would be difficult. There are several problems identifying how real the problem could be. Most people have little medical knowledge and even fewer question the cause of death. Also, even fewer people have autopsies performed. Then again, medical mistakes may lead to death with little relevance to an autopsy. Medical mistakes that lead to death may take a long time before death occurs and connections are made. There are professionals, such as attorneys and nurses, aware of these mistakes, but rarely get involved unless a lawsuit is involved. Recently, congress received enough complaints that a congressional investigation is being launched into the Joint Commission, as to its function in accreditation of hospitals. The fact that serious safety and sanitation issues have been identified by multiple individuals and groups raise awareness that our medical system isn't as perfect as the media would have us believe.

In summing up, over the last three years my companion had completed three surgical operations. The first operation was completed in the fall of 2013 at Rochester Hospital #2 for an intestinal obstruction and was found to be re-obstructed one year later. The re-obstruction probably occurred during the first two weeks following surgery and had nothing to do with the actual surgery. Instead, poor aftercare of "third spacing" that allowed excessive fluid to accumulate in body cavities was the cause of surgical failure.

Then, in the winter of 2014, one year later, the second surgical operation required to correct the first operation for intestinal re-obstruction was completed at Cleveland Hospital #4. During the fall of 2013 and most of 2014, TPN and antibiotics had kept Terry alive despite her becoming re-obstructed. She had been in and out of hospitals constantly for much of that time. Later it was discovered the first intestinal obstruction surgery had failed. Then re-obstruction surgery at Cleveland Hospital #4 in the fall of 2014 was successful, as a result of proper control of "third spacing". The following year 2015 was a healthy year for Terry.

Then, as of January 1st 2016, changes in Obama Care and Medicare resulted in Terry losing her access to TPN. That decision resulted in her suffering severe malnutrition and over whelming infections in the early months of 2016. These infections invaded her cervical spine and eyes, resulting in multiple eye surgeries and heavy doses of antibiotics were used to get the infections under control. These infections lingered however, and in November 2016, she redeveloped a lumbar spinal abscess. Her final surgical procedure for a spinal abscess was completed at Cleveland Hospital #4 in December 2016.

Much of her lengthy stays at Rochester Hospital #2 and Cleveland Hospital #4 were associated with the aftercare condition termed "third spacing". Her low protein albumin levels, coupled with too much administration of intravenous fluid, resulted in her arms, legs, and torso being severely swollen. It was necessary for her to ingest high quality protein in order to accumulate enough blood protein, albumin to keep fluid within her circulatory system. In the fall of 2014, at Cleveland Hospital #4, it took only 7 to 10 days of adequate meals to keep "third spacing" from getting out of control. By properly controlling intravenous fluid therapy and diuretic use, on an as needed basis, her "third spacing" had been minimized.

When Terry had been immobilized with a rectal hose and

administered excessive fluid therapy, she could neither feel like eating or exercising. These two essential functions were necessary for recovery from "third spacing". Unfortunately, a different group of doctors at the same hospital refused her diuretics, while nearly drowning her in intravenous therapy. Fluid therapy serves a useful purpose in blood pressure, hydration and electrolyte maintenance. However, intravenous therapy if improperly administered can result in life ending complications.

Over time, Terry had learned too much intravenous fluid was not good for her. At other hospitals, if she began noticing swelling in her arms and legs, she would inform doctors to stop fluid and would request a diuretic. Unfortunately, at Cleveland Hospital #4 twenty-four hours after her recovery, Dilaudid had been administered for pain resulting in her delirium. Delirium made it impossible for her to make rational decisions affecting her own welfare. Delirium also prevented her from reacting to her circumstances of so much intravenous fluids being pumped into her veins. Two crucial doctor mistakes, the use of a rectal hose and too much intravenous fluid quickly overwhelmed her.

Which leads me to a very important question. Should doctors and hospitals have the RIGHT to use drugs that remove the patient from their conscious environment, especially without permission from family or a medical power of attorney? Many of the pain drugs are opioids and their side effects of delirium do occur.

What is truly amazing is that, following her spinal abscess surgery, a patient such as Terry possessing all the serious medical issues, as short bowel disease, kidney transplant, and the recent spinal abscess, Cleveland Hospital #4 did NOT immediately place her in an intensive care unit. Rather, they sent her to a routine recovery unit. Even after she had suffered from delirium and doctors had "third spaced" her for that week following her surgery, she still was NOT sent to an intensive care unit. Finally, on Christmas

Eve, when Terry exhibited neurological symptoms preceding her seizure, she again was NOT admitted to an intensive care unit.

The medical literature can attest to all the medical complications associated with the condition termed "third spacing". Yet I, as a veterinarian, had never heard of this condition until my companion was faced with it. In questioning colleagues in my profession, they also considered this a non-issue. When faced with such an event where the patient visibly appeared swollen and overhydrated from too much intravenous fluid, simply less fluid was delivered or completely removed. Diuretics are rarely needed. Why is it then, that doctors find it necessary to administer such volumes of intravenous fluids, especially to protein deficient patients, or patients that have had a kidney transplant? "Third spacing" complications can place lives in jeopardy? Much like water intoxication, too much of anything can result in death. As a matter of fact, many of the same symptoms present in water intoxication are the same as "third spacing".

In summation, there are two hospital misconceptions that led to my companion's death. There are differences in opinion among both doctors and hospitals for treatment options concerned with "third spacing". The first misconception is that "third spacing" is alright. The patient is administered so much intravenous fluid so as to exhibit shortness of breath. Then, the patient is sent to an intensive care unit to have body cavities drained by needles. This practice creates complications well documented that need not occur. By simply controlling how much intravenous fluid is given, these patients do fine, as illustrated in my book. This misconception is based on the belief that pressure deficits may materialize which may actually be the opposite. It is reasonable to reduce intravenous fluid or discontinue its use, and use diuretics as needed if necessary.

The second misconception by nephrologists is that diuretics are SO TOXIC that a kidney transplant patient might lose their one kidney from the drug's use. Therefore, it is justified for these doctors to continue "third spacing" these patients until the patient is short of breath from fluid accumulation in their chest cavities. Then, the patient is delivered to the intensive care unit for fluid removal by needles and, guess what, all of a sudden diuretics are OK. I guess it's Ok to lose a life versus the unjustified lack of use of diuretics in "third spacing". Also, what about the complications from the use of needles in body cavities.

Over years I have used diuretics in veterinary medicine routinely and have never evidenced the extreme toxicity that had been related to me by doctors, while attempting to assist Terry. While in practice, I may not have had the option of using diuretics on kidney transplants, but I used diuretics often in heart patients and other conditions that were burdened by excess fluid. Even if these doctors and hospitals claim were even remotely correct, hospitals can monitor blood work on a daily basis for any changes that might occur to the kidney. In hypoproteinemic patients, adjustments with fluid and diuretics can control "third spacing. Had diuretics been used earlier in Terry's treatment for "third spacing", complications would not have occurred, and diuretic use would have been minimal. LACK of early intervention resulted in far more diuretics being administered to that one kidney. Once fluid continued to accumulate, doctors in the intensive care units didn't seem to worry much about diuretics and her one kidney. Apparently, diuretic use in transplant patients is considered a last resort for SOME doctors but not others. For those doctors and hospitals concerned about kidney transplants losing their one kidney due to diuretic use, they should reconsider. Terry didn't lose her kidney from diuretics, she lost her kidney due to complications from NOT using these drugs.

Over the last three years, Terry's insurance companies and Medicare paid out between two and three million dollars to doctors and hospitals for her care. During that time period, Terry, Snoot, and I had traveled thousands of miles to and from multiple hospitals in our attempt to find some medical resolution that never transpired. I can't help wondering how different Terry's life might have been had her first surgical procedure been successful. Then again, Terry with all her serious medical conditions at Cleveland Hospital #4 never was admitted to an intensive care unit. Very SAD! Terry and I had truly experienced "FIVE HOSPITALS AND A MEDICAL JOURNEY THROUGH HELL".

About the Author

Roger E Gussett was born in Columbus, Ohio. His parents divorced at an early age, and the family moved to a small 75-acre farm to live with his grandparents. The rural setting resulted in Roger's interest in Veterinary Medicine. In 1968, Roger graduated from The Ohio State University Veterinary College and then joined the Army Veterinary Corp for two years. Following service, Roger entered private practice to form Airport Animal Hospital, specializing in small animal medicine. He recently retired following 40+ years of service. Roger's interest in becoming an author was piqued following 3 years of shadowing the human medical field of his companion of 30 years that was placed on life support following unusual circumstances.

Made in the USA
Columbia, SC
20 August 2024